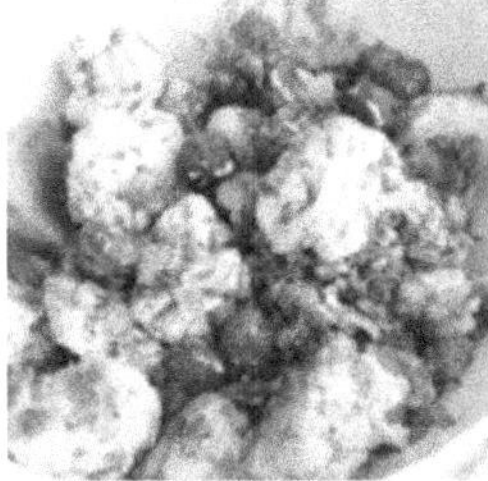

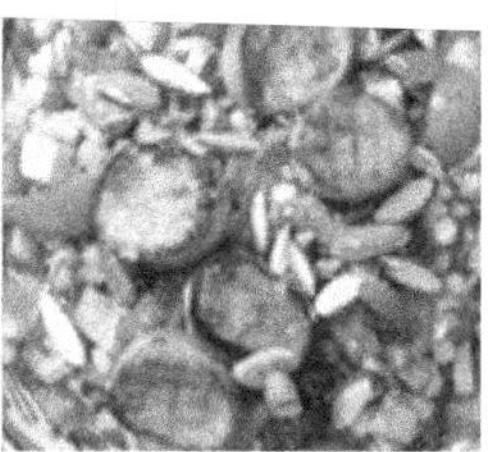

Dr. Josephine Samuel

5 IN 1 BOOK

The RHEUMATOID ARTHRITIS Recipe Cookbook

150 EASY AND DELICIOUS RECIPES TO REDUCE INFLAMMATION AND BOOST YOUR IMMUNE SYSTEM

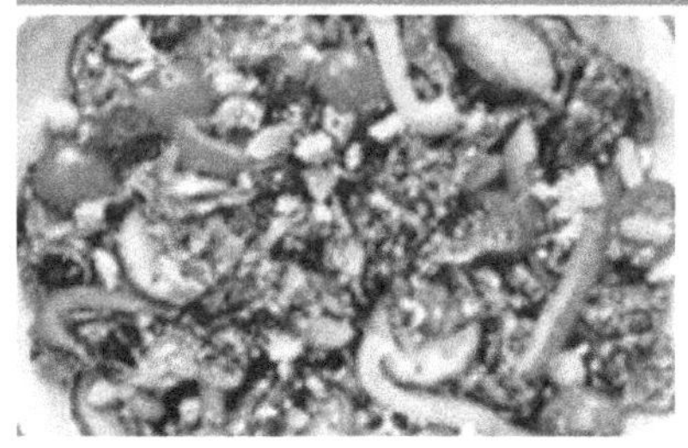

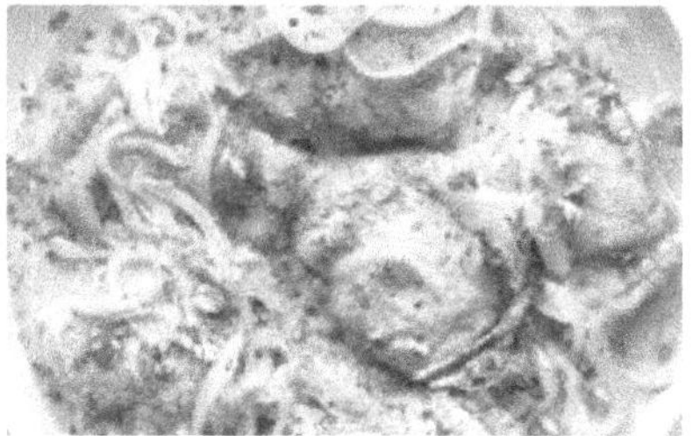

Rheumatoid Arthritis

Recipe

Cookbook

5 IN 1 MANUSCRIPT

- BREAKFAST
- LUNCH
- DINNER
- SNACK
- DESSERT
- JUICE
- SMOOTHIES

150 ANTI-INFLAMMATORY RECIPES (INCLUDING BREAKFAST, LUNCH, DINNER, DESSERTS, SMOOTHIES AND JUICE) TO MANAGE JOINTS AND FIGHT FATIGUE

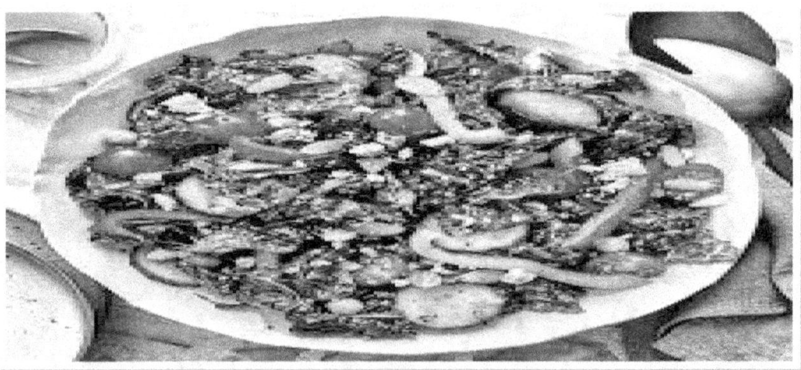

DR. JOSEPHINE SAMUEL

RHEUMATOID ARTHRITIS RECIPE COOKBOOK

Dear Valued Readers,

I am truly grateful for your support and for choosing my Rheumatoid Arthritis Recipe Cookbook to embark on your journey towards better health and well-being. Your decision to prioritize your health is commendable, and I'm thrilled to be a part of your wellness journey.

Living with rheumatoid arthritis can present its challenges, but it's also an opportunity to explore new ways of nourishing your body and embracing a lifestyle that supports your overall health. My cookbook is designed with your needs in mind, offering delicious and nutritious recipes that not only taste great but also help alleviate symptoms and promote joint health.

As you flip through the pages of my cookbook, you'll find a diverse array of recipes carefully crafted to be both flavorful and beneficial for managing rheumatoid arthritis. From hearty soups and comforting stews to vibrant salads and satisfying main courses, each recipe is thoughtfully curated to incorporate ingredients known for their anti-inflammatory properties and joint-friendly benefits.

I understand that eating well is not only about fueling your body but also about enjoying the experience of preparing and sharing meals with loved ones. That's why my cookbook is filled with recipes that are not only easy to follow but also a joy to create, whether you're cooking for yourself or for a gathering of friends and family.

I would like to express my heartfelt gratitude to everyone who contributed to the creation of this cookbook, from our talented chefs and nutrition experts to the individuals who shared their personal stories and insights. Your expertise and dedication have truly made this cookbook a labor of love, and I'm excited to share it with you.

Finally, I want to extend a special thank you to my readers. Your trust and support mean the world to me, and I hope that my cookbook becomes a valuable resource in your kitchen and on your journey towards better health.

With warmest regards,

Dr. Josephine Samuel

Dr. Josephine Samuel

This book is dedicated to all those
struggling with Arthritis

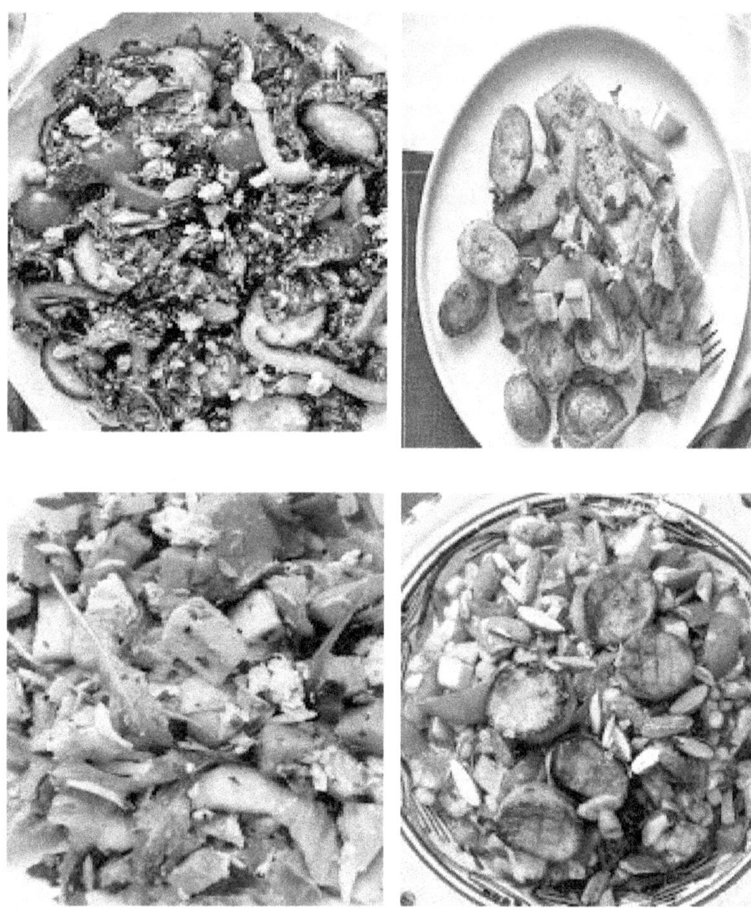

<u>BOOK 3</u>

<u>**RHEUMATOID ARTHRITIS DINNER RECIPES**</u>

BOOK 5

RHEUMATOID ARTHRITIS JUICE AND SMOOTHIE RECIPES

INTRODUCTION

Are you tired of the relentless pain, stiffness, and limitations that rheumatoid arthritis has imposed on your life? Are you ready to break free from its grip and reclaim the vibrant, pain-free existence you deserve?

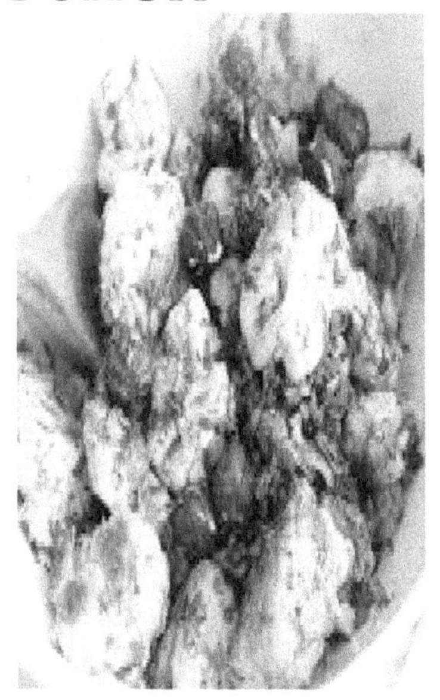

LOOK NO FURTHER RHEUMATOID ARTHRITIS RECIPE COOKBOOK IS YOUR TICKET TO LASTING RELIEF!

★ Break Free from the Chains of Pain! ★

❋ Uncover the groundbreaking strategies and insights that have empowered countless individuals to not only manage but conquer rheumatoid arthritis.

💪 Say goodbye to agony and discomfort as you explore natural, science-backed remedies that provide lasting relief.

🚀 Reclaim your life and rediscover the joy of simple pleasures as you experience increased mobility and energy.

🌟 Your Path to Freedom Begins NOW!

🔥 Rheumatoid Arthritis Recipe Cookbook is your key to a pain-free, revitalized life

Don't allow rheumatoid arthritis to dictate your life any longer.

Click the "Buy Now" button and embark on your transformative journey with Rheumatoid Arthritis Recipe Cookbook

🏆 Join the ranks of those who have overcome the odds, defied pain, and embraced vitality. Your relief is within reach, and it starts with this powerful book! 🏆

HOW TO SCAN THE ABOVE BARCODE

- Open the Camera app on your mobile phone.

- Position the barcode within the camera frame.

- Focus the camera on the barcode and capture the image.

- Wait for the camera to recognize and process the barcode.

- View all the books I have written for your healthy eating

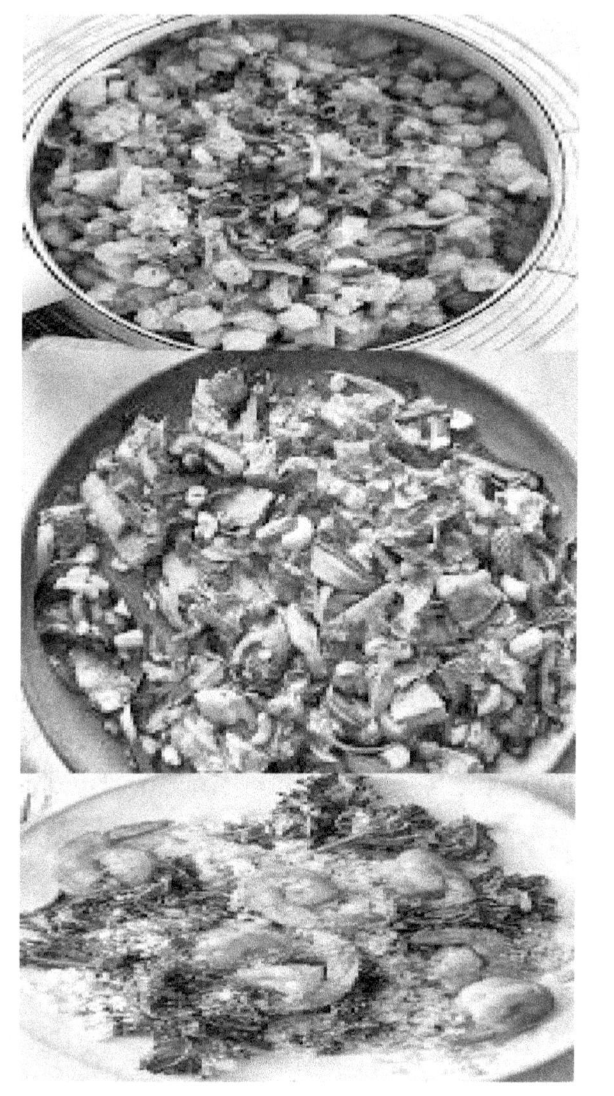

RHEUMATOID ARTHRITIS

An autoimmune illness that primarily affects the joints but can also affect other sections of the body is rheumatoid arthritis (RA). The tissue that lines the joints, the synovium, becomes inflamed, which causes joint pain, swelling, and stiffness. Over time, RA can harm the bones and cartilage in the joints, resulting in deformities and function loss. Even though there is no known treatment for RA, early detection and the right care can help control symptoms and avoid permanent joint damage.

Rheumatoid arthritis types include:

1. The most typical form of RA is seropositive, when blood tests reveal the presence of anti-cyclic citrullinated peptide (anti-CCP) antibodies and/or rheumatoid factor (RF).

2. Seronegative RA is a form of RA in which patients lack RF or anti-CCP antibodies that can be found in blood samples.

CAUSES OF RHEUMATOID ARTHRITIS

Although the precise etiology of RA is unknown, it is thought to be the result of a mix of immune system, genetic, and environmental factors. Exposure to specific environmental stimuli, such as infections or smoking, may cause individuals with a genetic predisposition to experience immune system activation and an autoimmune reaction that attacks the synovium.

SYMPTOMS OF RHEUMATOID ARTHRITIS

1. Joint Pain and Swelling: Ongoing joint pain, swelling, and tenderness that frequently affects many joints at once.

2. Morning stiffness: Joint stiffness, especially in the morning or following periods of inactivity.

3. Fatigue: The body's immunological reaction and the effects of inflammation cause you to feel fatigued and low on energy.

4. Joint Deformities: RA may eventually result in joint deformities, which can impair mobility and function.

5. Flares and Remissions: RA symptoms can fluctuate, with times when the disease is more active (called flares) and times when it is less active (called remissions).

6. Fever, weight loss, and a general feeling of being poorly are possible symptoms for some people.

RHEUMATOID ARTHRITIS MANAGEMENT AND TREATMENT

Although there is no known cure for RA, a number of therapeutic modalities work to reduce inflammation, manage symptoms, and guard against joint deterioration. Based on the severity of the condition, general health, and individual preferences, treatment strategies are frequently tailored.

TYPICAL FORMS OF TREATMENTS FOR RHEUMATOID ARTHRITIS

Medications: To lessen inflammation and limit the progression of RA, physicians may give nonsteroidal anti-inflammatory medications (NSAIDs), disease-modifying antirheumatic drugs (DMARDs), and biologic treatments.

Physical treatment: Physical therapy can help reduce pain and avoid joint abnormalities while also enhancing joint flexibility, strength, and function.

Occupational therapy: Occupational therapists can offer tips on how to handle daily tasks and guard against too much stress on the joints.

Lifestyle changes: Adopting a balanced diet, engaging in regular exercise, managing stress, and getting enough sleep can all have a favorable effect on RA symptoms.

Joint Protection: Protecting the joints from future harm can be done by using assistive devices and avoiding recurrent joint stress.

Surgery: To improve joint function and relieve discomfort in extreme situations, joint replacement surgery may be explored.

To create a thorough treatment plan, people with RA must collaborate closely with a rheumatologist. People with rheumatoid arthritis can dramatically enhance their quality of life with early diagnosis and rapid treatment.

BOOK 1

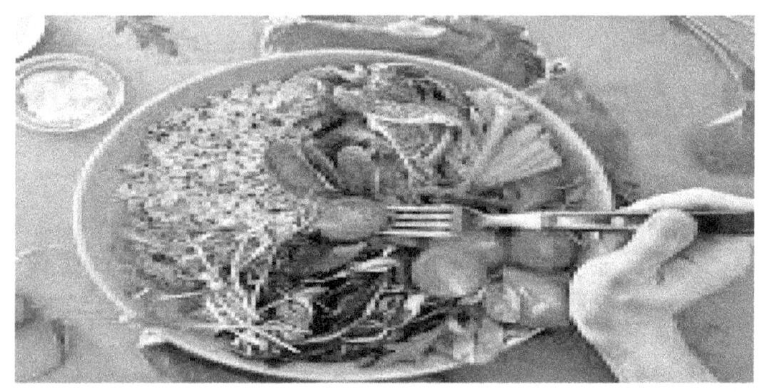

BREAKFAST DISHES FOR RHEUMATOID ARTHRITIS, ALONG WITH PREPARATION INSTRUCTIONS

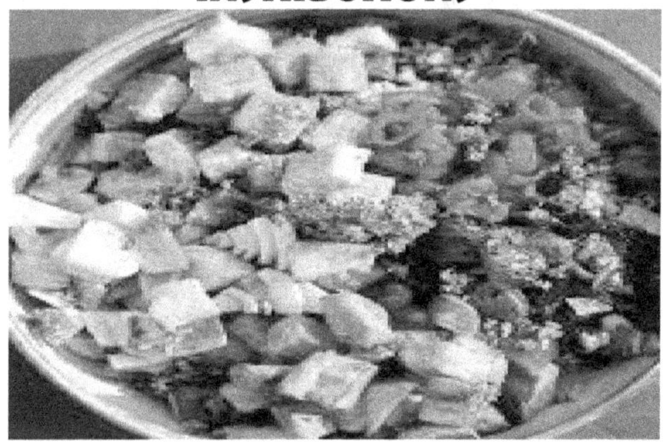

BREAKFAST DISHES FOR RHEUMATOID ARTHRITIS, ALONG WITH PREPARATION INSTRUCTIONS

Recipe 1

Mango-Turmeric Smoothie

Ingredients: Mango, turmeric, Greek yogurt, almond milk, honey, and chia seeds are the ingredients.

Instructions: Greek yogurt, mango, turmeric, almond milk, honey, and chia seeds should all be thoroughly blended.

Recipe 2

Breakfast bowl with quinoa

Almond milk, sliced bananas, mixed berries, cooked quinoa, and a sprinkle of honey are the ingredients.

Instructions: In a bowl, combine the cooked quinoa, almond milk, mixed berries, and banana slices. Add honey to the dish.

Recipe 3

Frittata with sweet potatoes and spinach

Ingredients: Sweet potatoes, spinach, eggs, onions, garlic, and olive oil are the ingredients.

Instructions: Cook spinach, onions, garlic, and sweet potatoes in olive oil. Pour beaten eggs over the vegetables. until done, bake.

Recipe 4

Toast with tomato and avocado

Avocado, cherry tomatoes, whole grain toast, olive oil, and balsamic vinegar are the ingredients.

Instructions: On the toast, mash the avocado. Add cherry tomatoes on top and drizzle with balsamic vinegar and olive oil.

Recipe 5

Blueberry Chia Pudding with Almonds

Ingredients: Chia seeds, almond milk, almond butter, blueberries, and a trace of maple syrup are the ingredients.

Mix the following ingredients in a jar: chia seeds, almond milk, almond butter, blueberries, and maple syrup. Overnight refrigerate.

Recipe 6

Vegetables and egg white omelette

Ingredients: Egg whites, diced bell peppers, mushrooms, spinach, onions, and a sprinkle of black pepper.

Instructions: Whisk egg whites and pour them into a non-stick pan. Add diced vegetables and cook until set.

Recipe 7

Cottage Cheese with Pineapple and Walnuts

Ingredients: Low-fat cottage cheese, diced pineapple, chopped walnuts, and a drizzle of honey.

Instructions: Combine cottage cheese, pineapple, and walnuts in a bowl. Drizzle with honey.

Recipe 8

Banana Walnut Muffins

Ingredients: Whole wheat flour, mashed bananas, chopped walnuts, Greek yogurt, eggs, and honey.

Instructions: Mix all the ingredients in a bowl. Pour the batter into muffin cups and bake until golden.

Recipe 9

Coconut Chia Seed Porridge

Ingredients: Chia seeds, coconut milk, shredded coconut, sliced almonds, and fresh berries.

Instructions: Mix chia seeds, coconut milk, shredded coconut, and sliced almonds. Refrigerate overnight. Top with fresh berries before serving.

Recipe 10

Pumpkin Spice Overnight Oats

Ingredients: Rolled oats, pumpkin puree, almond milk, maple syrup, pumpkin pie spice, and chopped pecans.

Instructions: Mix oats, pumpkin puree, almond milk, maple syrup, and pumpkin pie spice in a jar. Refrigerate overnight. Top with chopped pecans before serving.

Recipe 11

Savory Breakfast Burrito

Ingredients: Scrambled eggs, black beans, diced avocado, salsa, and whole wheat tortilla.

Instructions: Fill the tortilla with scrambled eggs, black beans, diced avocado, and salsa. Roll it up into a burrito.

Recipe 12

Mango Coconut Chia Pudding

Ingredients: Chia seeds, coconut milk, ripe mango, shredded coconut, and honey.

Instructions: Blend mango and coconut milk until smooth. Mix with chia seeds and honey. Refrigerate overnight.

Recipe 13

Apple Cinnamon Overnight Oats

Ingredients: Rolled oats, diced apples, almond milk, cinnamon, and a drizzle of maple syrup.

Instructions: Mix oats, apples, almond milk, cinnamon, and maple syrup in a jar. Refrigerate overnight.

Recipe 14

Yogurt Parfait with Berries and Granola

Ingredients: Greek yogurt, mixed berries, granola, and a drizzle of honey.

Instructions: Layer Greek yogurt, mixed berries, and granola in a glass. Drizzle with honey.

Recipe 15

Chickpea Flour Pancakes

Ingredients: Chickpea flour, water, diced bell peppers, chopped spinach, and a pinch of turmeric.

Instructions: Mix chickpea flour, water, bell peppers, spinach, and turmeric to make the batter. Cook in a non-stick pan until golden.

Recipe 16

Cherry Almond Smoothie Bowl

Ingredients: Frozen cherries, almond milk, almond butter, Greek yogurt, and sliced almonds.

Instructions: Blend cherries, almond milk, almond butter, and Greek yogurt until smooth. Pour into a bowl and top with sliced almonds.

Sesame Banana Toast

Ingredients: Whole grain toast, sliced bananas, tahini, and a sprinkle of sesame seeds.

Instructions: Spread tahini on the toast. Top with sliced bananas and sprinkle sesame seeds.

Berry Chia Seed Pudding

Ingredients: Chia seeds, almond milk, mixed berries, and a touch of honey.

Instructions: Mix chia seeds, almond milk, mixed berries, and honey in a jar. Refrigerate overnight.

Ingredients: Eggs, spinach, mushrooms, diced onions, and a pinch of black pepper.

Instructions: Whisk eggs and pour them into a non-stick pan. Add spinach, mushrooms, and onions. Cook until set.

Recipe 20

Peanut Butter Banana Smoothie

Ingredients: Ripe bananas, peanut butter, Greek yogurt, almond milk, and a drizzle of honey.

Instructions: Blend bananas, peanut butter, Greek yogurt, almond milk, and honey until smooth.

Recipe 21

Broccoli and Cheese Frittata

Ingredients: Broccoli florets, eggs, diced bell peppers, shredded cheese, and a sprinkle of black pepper.

Instructions: Steam broccoli until tender. Whisk eggs and pour them into a non-stick pan. Add steamed broccoli, bell peppers, and shredded cheese. Bake until set.

Recipe 22

Mixed Berry Chia Jam

Ingredients: Mixed berries, chia seeds, lemon juice, and a touch of honey.

Instructions: Mash berries and mix them with chia seeds, lemon juice, and honey. Let it sit for a few hours until it thickens.

Recipe 23

Cranberry Orange Overnight Oats

Ingredients: Rolled oats, dried cranberries, orange juice, almond milk, and a drizzle of maple syrup.

Instructions: Mix oats, cranberries, orange juice, almond milk, and maple syrup in a jar. Refrigerate overnight.

Recipe 24

Apricot Almond Smoothie

Ingredients: Fresh apricots, almond milk, almond butter, Greek yogurt, and a touch of honey.

Instructions: Blend apricots, almond milk, almond butter, Greek yogurt, and honey until smooth.

Recipe 25

Sweet Potato and Kale Breakfast Hash

Ingredients: Sweet potatoes, chopped kale, diced onions, garlic, and a pinch of paprika.

Instructions: Sauté sweet potatoes, kale, onions, and garlic in olive oil. Season with salt, pepper, and paprika. Cook until sweet potatoes are tender and kale is wilted.

NOTES

BOOK 2

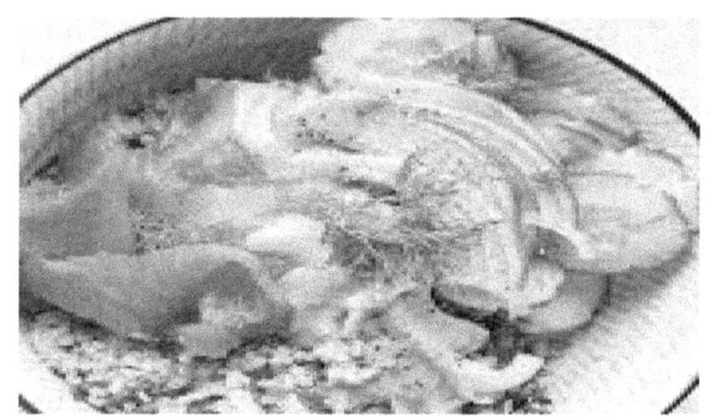

LUNCH RECIPES FOR RHEUMATOID ARTHRITIS, WITH PREPARATION INSTRUCTIONS

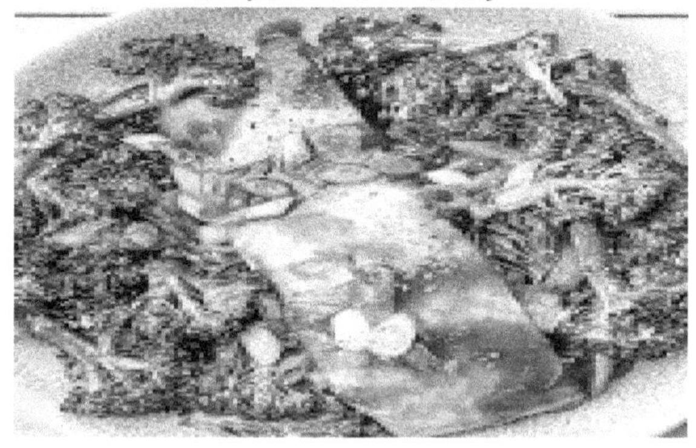

RHEUMATOID ARTHRITIS-
LUNCH RECIPES

Recipe 26

Grilled Chicken and Avocado Wrap

Ingredients: Grilled chicken breast, sliced avocado, mixed greens, diced tomatoes, whole wheat tortilla, and a dollop of Greek yogurt.

Instructions: Lay the tortilla flat and fill it with grilled chicken, avocado, mixed greens, tomatoes, and Greek yogurt. Roll it up into a wrap.

Recipe 27

Mediterranean Quinoa Bowl

Ingredients: Cooked quinoa, chopped cucumber, cherry tomatoes, Kalamata olives, feta cheese, lemon juice, olive oil, fresh oregano, salt, and pepper.

Instructions: Combine all the ingredients in a bowl and drizzle with lemon juice, olive oil, and season with oregano, salt, and pepper.

Recipe 28

Salmon and Quinoa Salad

Ingredients: Grilled salmon, cooked quinoa, diced bell peppers, diced red onion, chopped cilantro, lime juice, olive oil, salt, and pepper.

Instructions: Mix all the ingredients in a bowl and dress with lime juice, olive oil, salt, and pepper.

Recipe 29

Turkey and Avocado Lettuce Wraps

Ingredients: Sliced turkey breast, avocado slices, shredded carrots, shredded cabbage, lettuce leaves, and a drizzle of balsamic vinaigrette.

Instructions: Lay a lettuce leaf flat and fill it with turkey, avocado, carrots, and cabbage. Drizzle with balsamic vinaigrette and wrap it up.

Recipe 30

Roasted Vegetable Quinoa Bowl

Ingredients: Roasted vegetables (carrots, bell peppers, zucchini, broccoli), cooked quinoa, fresh spinach, lemon tahini dressing.

Instructions: Combine roasted vegetables, quinoa, and spinach in a bowl. Drizzle with lemon tahini dressing.

Recipe 31

Greek Chicken Pita

Ingredients: Grilled chicken breast, diced cucumber, diced tomatoes, feta cheese, Greek yogurt, whole wheat pita bread.

Instructions: Fill the pita bread with grilled chicken, cucumber, tomatoes, feta cheese, and Greek yogurt

Recipe 32

Tuna Salad Lettuce Wraps

Ingredients: Canned tuna, diced celery, diced red onion, diced pickles, Greek yogurt, Dijon mustard, lettuce leaves.

Instructions: Mix tuna, celery, onion, pickles, Greek yogurt, and mustard in a bowl. Spoon the mixture onto lettuce leaves and wrap.

Recipe 33

Cauliflower Rice Sushi Roll

Ingredients: Cauliflower rice, sliced cucumber, sliced avocado, sliced carrots, nori seaweed sheets, pickled ginger, low-sodium soy sauce.

Instructions: Lay a nori sheet flat and spread cauliflower rice over it. Add cucumber, avocado, and carrots. Roll it up tightly and slice into sushi rolls. Serve with pickled ginger and soy sauce.

Recipe 34

Greek Quinoa Stuffed Peppers

Ingredients: Cooked quinoa, diced tomatoes, Kalamata olives, feta cheese, fresh parsley, oregano, salt, and pepper, bell peppers.

Instructions: Preheat the oven to 375°F (190°C). Cut the tops off the bell peppers and remove seeds. Mix quinoa, tomatoes, olives, feta cheese, parsley, oregano, salt, and pepper. Stuff the peppers with the mixture and bake for about 20-25 minutes until peppers are tender.

Recipe 35

Asian Chicken Lettuce Wraps

Ingredients: Grilled chicken breast, shredded carrots, shredded cabbage, sliced scallions, chopped cilantro, low-sodium soy sauce, and lettuce leaves.

Instructions: Mix chicken, carrots, cabbage, scallions, cilantro, and soy sauce in a bowl. Spoon the mixture onto lettuce leaves and wrap.

Recipe 36

Mango Avocado Salad

Ingredients: Diced mango, diced avocado, mixed greens, sliced red onion, chopped cilantro, lime juice, and olive oil.

Instructions: Combine all the ingredients in a bowl and drizzle with lime juice and olive oil.

Recipe 37

Veggie Hummus Wrap

Ingredients: Hummus, sliced cucumber, sliced bell peppers, sliced tomatoes, shredded carrots, whole wheat tortilla.

Instructions: Spread hummus on the tortilla and fill it with cucumber, peppers, tomatoes, and carrots. Roll it up into a wrap.

Recipe 38

Quinoa and Black Bean Bowl

Ingredients: Cooked quinoa, canned black beans, diced bell peppers, diced red onion, chopped cilantro, lime juice, olive oil, salt, and pepper.

Instructions: Mix all the ingredients in a bowl and drizzle with lime juice, olive oil, salt, and pepper.

Recipe 39

Roasted Vegetable and Chickpea Salad

Ingredients: Roasted vegetables (sweet potatoes, Brussels sprouts, red onion), canned chickpeas, mixed greens, lemon-tahini dressing.

Instructions: Combine roasted vegetables, chickpeas, and mixed greens in a bowl. Drizzle with lemon-tahini dressing.

Tuna Avocado Salad

Ingredients: Canned tuna, diced avocado, diced red onion, chopped parsley, lemon juice, olive oil, salt, and pepper.

Instructions: Mix tuna, avocado, onion, parsley, lemon juice, olive oil, salt, and pepper in a bowl.

Spinach and Feta Stuffed Chicken Breast

Ingredients: Boneless, skinless chicken breasts, fresh spinach, crumbled feta cheese, garlic powder, salt, and pepper.

Instructions: Preheat the oven to 400°F (200°C). Cut a pocket in each chicken breast. Stuff each pocket with spinach and feta cheese. Sprinkle with garlic powder, salt, and pepper. Bake for about 20-25 minutes until chicken is cooked through.

Recipe 42

Mediterranean Chickpea Salad

Ingredients: Canned chickpeas, diced cucumber, cherry tomatoes, Kalamata olives, crumbled feta cheese, fresh parsley, lemon juice, olive oil, salt, and pepper.

Instructions: Mix all the ingredients in a bowl and drizzle with lemon juice, olive oil, salt, and pepper.

Recipe 43

Salmon and Cucumber Salad

Ingredients: Grilled salmon, sliced cucumber, cherry tomatoes, diced red onion, chopped dill, lemon juice, and olive oil.

Instructions: Combine all the ingredients in a bowl and drizzle with lemon juice and olive oil.

Mango Chicken Lettuce Wraps

Ingredients: Grilled chicken breast, diced mango, diced bell peppers, sliced scallions, chopped cilantro, lime juice, and lettuce leaves.

Instructions: Mix chicken, mango, peppers, scallions, cilantro, and lime juice in a bowl. Spoon the mixture onto lettuce leaves and wrap.

Egg Salad Stuffed Avocado

Ingredients: Hard-boiled eggs, diced celery, diced red onion, chopped dill, Greek yogurt, Dijon mustard, ripe avocados.

Instructions: Mash hard-boiled eggs and mix with celery, onion, dill, Greek yogurt, and mustard. Cut avocados in half and remove the pit. Stuff the avocado halves with the egg salad.

Recipe 46

Lemon Garlic Shrimp and Asparagus

Ingredients: Shrimp, asparagus spears, minced garlic, lemon juice, olive oil, salt, and pepper.

Instructions: Preheat the oven to 400°F (200°C). Toss shrimp and asparagus with garlic, lemon juice, olive oil, salt, and pepper. Arrange on a baking sheet and bake for about 10-12 minutes until shrimp is cooked through.

Recipe 47

Cauliflower Rice Burrito Bowl

Ingredients: Cauliflower rice, black beans, diced bell peppers, diced avocado, salsa, and a dollop of Greek yogurt.

Instructions: Steam cauliflower rice until tender. Mix cauliflower rice, black beans, peppers, avocado, and salsa in a bowl. Top with Greek yogurt.

Recipe 48

Tofu and Veggie Stir-Fry

Ingredients: Firm tofu, mixed stir-fry vegetables, low-sodium soy sauce, sesame oil, and cooked brown rice.

Instructions: Cut tofu into cubes. Sauté tofu and vegetables in sesame oil until cooked. Add soy sauce and serve over brown rice.

Recipe 49

Chicken and Vegetable Lettuce Wraps

Ingredients: Grilled chicken breast, mixed stir-fry vegetables, low-sodium soy sauce, and lettuce leaves.

Instructions: Sauté chicken and vegetables in a non-stick pan. Add soy sauce and spoon the mixture onto lettuce leaves. Wrap and enjoy!

Recipe 50

Quinoa and Chickpea Salad

Ingredients: Cooked quinoa, canned chickpeas, diced cucumber, cherry tomatoes, fresh parsley, lemon juice, olive oil, salt, and pepper.

Instructions: Mix all the ingredients in a bowl and toss with lemon juice, olive oil, salt, and pepper.

These lunch recipes are packed with nutritious ingredients that are not only delicious but also suitable for individuals with rheumatoid arthritis. Enjoy these flavorful and satisfying meals while supporting your overall health and well-being.

NOTES

BOOK 3

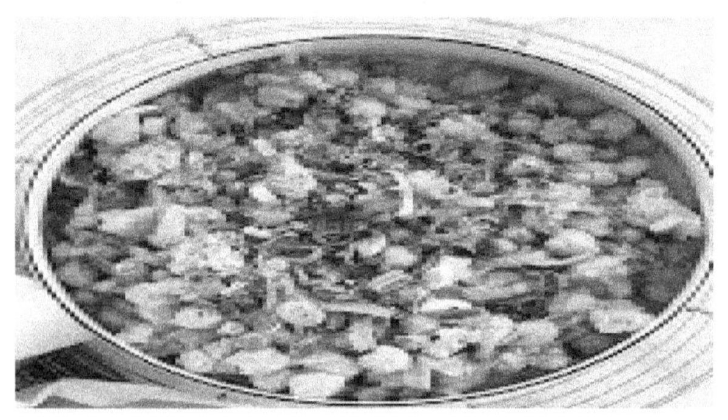

DINNER RECIPES FOR RHEUMATOID ARTHRITIS, WITH PREPARATION INSTRUCTIONS

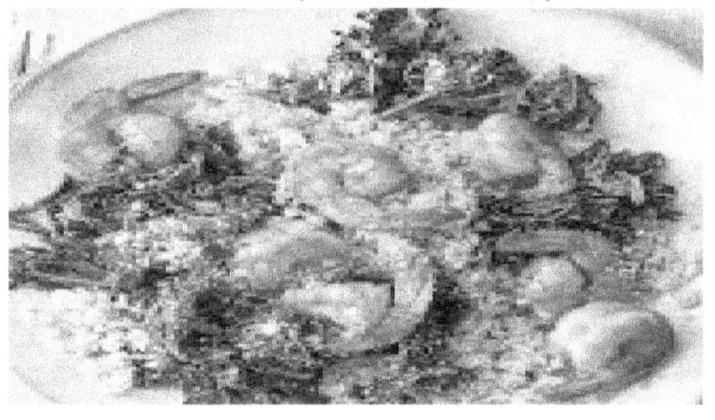

RHEUMATOID ARTHRITIS-DINNER RECIPES

Recipe 51

Baked Salmon with Roasted Vegetables

Ingredients: Salmon fillet, mixed vegetables (carrots, bell peppers, zucchini), olive oil, lemon juice, garlic, salt, and pepper.

Instructions: Place the salmon on a baking sheet. Toss the mixed vegetables with olive oil, lemon juice, garlic, salt, and pepper. Roast both in the oven until cooked.

Recipe 52

Lemon Herb Grilled Chicken

Ingredients: Chicken breast, lemon juice, olive oil, garlic, dried herbs (rosemary, thyme, oregano), salt, and pepper.

Instructions: Marinate the chicken in lemon juice, olive oil, garlic, herbs, salt, and pepper. Grill until fully cooked.

Recipe 53

Vegetarian Stuffed Bell Peppers

Ingredients: Bell peppers, cooked quinoa, black beans, diced tomatoes, diced onions, shredded cheese (optional), taco seasoning, salt, and pepper.

Instructions: Cut the tops off the bell peppers and remove the seeds. Mix cooked quinoa, black beans, tomatoes, onions, cheese, and taco seasoning. Stuff the peppers and bake until tender.

Recipe 54

Sesame Ginger Tofu Stir-Fry

Ingredients: Firm tofu, mixed stir-fry vegetables, low-sodium soy sauce, sesame oil, ginger, garlic, and cooked brown rice.

Instructions: Cut tofu into cubes and sauté with vegetables in sesame oil, ginger, and garlic. Add soy sauce and serve over brown rice.

Recipe 55

Mediterranean Chickpea and Quinoa Salad

Ingredients: Cooked quinoa, canned chickpeas, diced cucumbers, cherry tomatoes, Kalamata olives, feta cheese, fresh parsley, lemon juice, olive oil, salt, and pepper.

Instructions: Mix all the ingredients in a bowl and drizzle with lemon juice, olive oil, salt, and pepper.

Recipe 56

Baked Chicken with Sweet Potato Fries

Ingredients: Chicken thighs, sweet potatoes, olive oil, paprika, garlic powder, salt, and pepper.

Instructions: Rub chicken with olive oil, paprika, garlic powder, salt, and pepper. Bake in the oven along with sweet potato fries until fully cooked.

Recipe 57

Spinach and Feta Stuffed Portobello Mushrooms

Ingredients: Portobello mushrooms, fresh spinach, crumbled feta cheese, garlic, salt, and pepper.

Instructions: Preheat the oven to 400°F (200°C). Remove the stems from the mushrooms and scrape out the gills. Sauté spinach and garlic until wilted. Stuff the mushrooms with the spinach mixture and top with feta cheese. Bake until mushrooms are tender.

Recipe 58

Black Bean and Quinoa Burrito Bowl

Ingredients: Cooked quinoa, canned black beans, diced bell peppers, diced avocado, salsa, and a dollop of Greek yogurt.

Instructions: Mix quinoa, black beans, peppers, avocado, and salsa in a bowl. Top with Greek yogurt.

Stuffed Zucchini Boats

Ingredients: Zucchini, ground turkey, diced tomatoes, diced onions, garlic, Italian seasoning, salt, and pepper.

Instructions: Preheat the oven to 375°F (190°C). Cut the zucchini in half lengthwise and scoop out the insides. Sauté ground turkey with tomatoes, onions, garlic, seasoning, salt, and pepper. Stuff the zucchini with the mixture and bake until zucchini is tender.

Balsamic Glazed Pork Chops

Ingredients: Pork chops, balsamic vinegar, honey, garlic, dried thyme, salt, and pepper.

Instructions: Mix balsamic vinegar, honey, garlic, thyme, salt, and pepper. Marinate the pork chops in the mixture. Grill or bake until fully cooked.

Recipe 61

Shrimp and Broccoli Stir-Fry

Ingredients: Shrimp, broccoli florets, low-sodium soy sauce, garlic, ginger, sesame oil, and cooked brown rice.

Instructions: Sauté shrimp and broccoli in sesame oil, garlic, and ginger. Add soy sauce and serve over brown rice.

Recipe 62

Lemon Herb Baked Chicken Thighs

Ingredients: Chicken thighs, lemon juice, olive oil, garlic, dried herbs (rosemary, thyme, oregano), salt, and pepper.

Instructions: Marinate the chicken in lemon juice, olive oil, garlic, herbs, salt, and pepper. Bake until fully cooked.

Recipe 63

Cauliflower Rice with Garlic Shrimp

Ingredients: Cauliflower rice, shrimp, garlic, lemon juice, olive oil, parsley, salt, and pepper.

Instructions: Sauté shrimp with garlic, lemon juice, olive oil, parsley, salt, and pepper. Serve over cauliflower rice.

Recipe 64

Turkey Meatball Lettuce Wraps

Ingredients: Ground turkey, diced bell peppers, diced onions, garlic, egg, breadcrumbs, lettuce leaves, and a drizzle of Greek yogurt.

Instructions: Mix ground turkey, peppers, onions, garlic, egg, and breadcrumbs. Form into meatballs and bake until cooked. Serve in lettuce wraps and drizzle with Greek yogurt.

Baked Cod with Lemon and Herbs

Ingredients: Cod fillets, lemon juice, olive oil, garlic, dried herbs (parsley, dill, thyme), salt, and pepper.

Instructions: Preheat the oven to 375°F (190°C). Place cod fillets on a baking sheet. Mix lemon juice, olive oil, garlic, herbs, salt, and pepper. Pour the mixture over the fish. Bake until fully cooked.

Chickpea and Sweet Potato Curry

Ingredients: Canned chickpeas, sweet potatoes, diced tomatoes, diced onions, garlic, curry powder, coconut milk, and cooked basmati rice.

Instructions: Sauté sweet potatoes, onions, and garlic. Add chickpeas, tomatoes, curry powder, and coconut milk. Simmer until sweet potatoes are tender. Serve over basmati rice.

Zucchini Noodles with Pesto and Cherry Tomatoes

Ingredients: Zucchini noodles, homemade or store-bought pesto, cherry tomatoes, and grated Parmesan cheese.

Instructions: Sauté zucchini noodles until slightly tender. Toss with pesto and cherry tomatoes. Top with grated Parmesan cheese.

Stuffed Bell Peppers with Quinoa and Lentils

Ingredients: Bell peppers, cooked quinoa, cooked lentils, diced tomatoes, diced onions, garlic, cumin, paprika, salt, and pepper.

Instructions: Cut the tops off the bell peppers and remove the seeds. Mix quinoa, lentils, tomatoes, onions, garlic, cumin, paprika, salt, and pepper. Stuff the peppers and bake until tender.

Recipe 69

Moroccan Chickpea and Vegetable Stew

Ingredients: Canned chickpeas, diced carrots, diced sweet potatoes, diced bell peppers, diced onions, garlic, cumin, coriander, cinnamon, vegetable broth.

Instructions: Sauté onions and garlic. Add carrots, sweet potatoes, bell peppers, spices, and vegetable broth. Simmer until vegetables are tender. Add chickpeas and continue to simmer.

Recipe 70

Salmon and Quinoa Stuffed Bell Peppers

Ingredients: Bell peppers, cooked quinoa, grilled salmon, diced tomatoes, diced onions, garlic, lemon juice, fresh dill, salt, and pepper.

Instructions: Cut the tops off the bell peppers and remove the seeds. Mix quinoa, salmon, tomatoes, onions, garlic, lemon juice, dill, salt, and pepper. Stuff the peppers and bake until tender.

Lemon Garlic Shrimp Pasta

Ingredients: Shrimp, whole wheat spaghetti, minced garlic, lemon juice, olive oil, fresh parsley, salt, and pepper.

Instructions: Cook the spaghetti according to the package instructions. Sauté shrimp with garlic, lemon juice, olive oil, parsley, salt, and pepper. Toss with cooked pasta.

Eggplant Parmesan

Ingredients: Eggplant slices, marinara sauce, shredded mozzarella cheese, grated Parmesan cheese, dried oregano, dried basil.

Instructions: Preheat the oven to 375°F (190°C). Layer eggplant slices with marinara sauce, mozzarella, Parmesan, oregano, and basil. Repeat the layers. Bake until cheese is melted and bubbly.

Recipe 73

Cilantro Lime Shrimp Tacos

Ingredients: Shrimp, corn tortillas, shredded cabbage, diced tomatoes, chopped cilantro, lime juice, Greek yogurt.

Instructions: Sauté shrimp with lime juice. Warm the corn tortillas. Fill each tortilla with shrimp, cabbage, tomatoes, cilantro, and a dollop of Greek yogurt.

Recipe 74

Garlic Herb Baked Pork Tenderloin

Ingredients: Pork tenderloin, minced garlic, dried herbs (rosemary, thyme, oregano), olive oil, salt, and pepper.

Instructions: Preheat the oven to 400°F (200°C). Rub the pork tenderloin with minced garlic, herbs, olive oil, salt, and pepper. Bake until fully cooked.

Recipe 75

Cauliflower and Chickpea Curry

Ingredients: Cauliflower florets, canned chickpeas, diced tomatoes, diced onions, garlic, curry powder, coconut milk, and cooked basmati rice.

Instructions: Sauté onions and garlic. Add cauliflower, chickpeas, tomatoes, curry powder, and coconut milk. Simmer until cauliflower is tender. Serve over basmati rice.

These dinner recipes are not only healthy and flavorful but also rich in nutrients that are beneficial for individuals with rheumatoid arthritis. Enjoy these delicious meals while taking care of your health and well-being.

NOTES

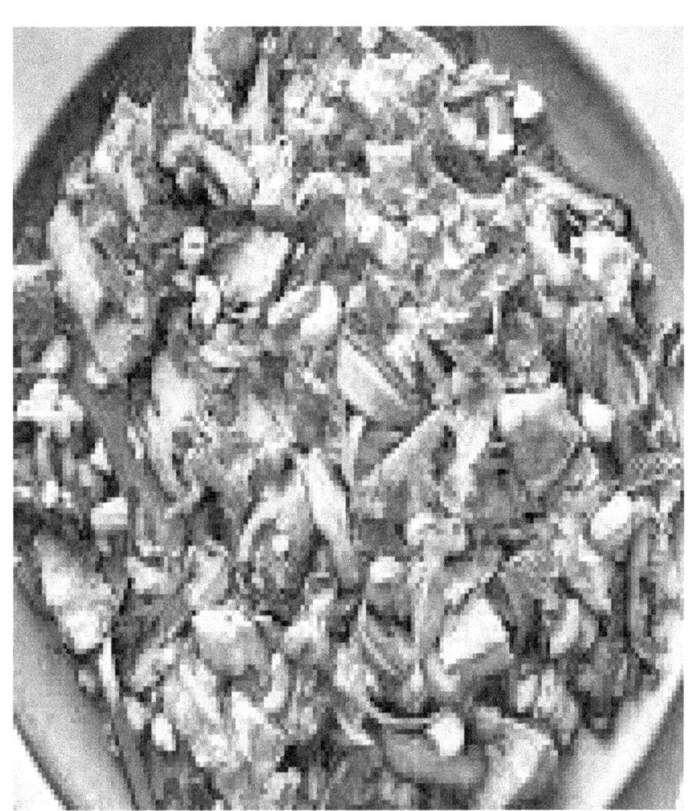

BOOK 4

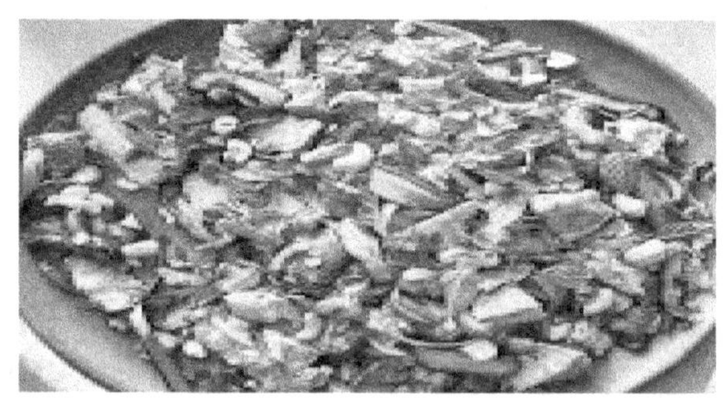

SNACKS AND DESSERT RECIPES FOR RHEUMATOID ARTHRITIS, WITH PREPARATION INSTRUCTIONS

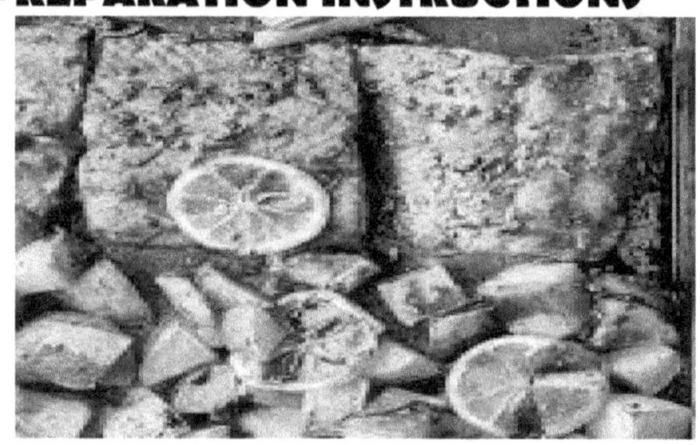

RHEUMATOID ARTHRITIS- SNACKS AND DESSERT RECIPES

Snacks

Recipe 76

Greek Yogurt Parfait

Ingredients: Greek yogurt, honey, granola, mixed berries.

Instructions: Layer Greek yogurt, honey, granola, and mixed berries in a glass.

Recipe 77

Celery Sticks with Hummus

Ingredients: Celery sticks, hummus.

Instructions: Dip celery sticks in hummus.

Carrot Sticks with Guacamol

Ingredients: Carrot sticks, guacamole.

Instructions: Dip carrot sticks in guacamole.

Recipe 78

Trail Mix

Ingredients: Almonds, walnuts, dried cranberries, dark chocolate chips.

Instructions: Mix all the ingredients together.

Recipe 79

Cherry Tomato and Mozzarella Skewers

Ingredients: Cherry tomatoes, mozzarella balls, fresh basil leaves, balsamic glaze.

Instructions: Skewer cherry tomatoes, mozzarella balls, and basil leaves. Drizzle with balsamic glaze.

Recipe 80

Cucumber Slices with Tzatziki Sauce

Ingredients: Cucumber slices, tzatziki sauce.

Instructions: Dip cucumber slices in tzatziki sauce.

Recipe 81

Sliced Apple with Almond Butter

Ingredients: Apple slices, almond butter.

Instructions: Spread almond butter on apple slices.

Recipe 82

Rice Cakes with Avocado

Ingredients: Rice cakes, avocado slices, sea salt, and black pepper.

Instructions: Top rice cakes with avocado slices. Sprinkle with sea salt and black pepper.

Recipe 83

Mixed Berries Smoothie

Ingredients: Mixed berries (strawberries, blueberries, raspberries), almond milk, Greek yogurt, honey.

Instructions: Blend all the ingredients until smooth.

Recipe 84

Zucchini Chips

Ingredients: Zucchini slices, olive oil, paprika, salt, and pepper.

Instructions: Toss zucchini slices with olive oil, paprika, salt, and pepper. Bake until crispy.

Recipe 85

Edamame

Ingredients: Frozen edamame, sea salt.

Instructions: Steam edamame and sprinkle with sea salt.

Kale Chips

Ingredients: Fresh kale leaves, olive oil, nutritional yeast, garlic powder, salt, and pepper.

Instructions: Toss kale leaves with olive oil, nutritional yeast, garlic powder, salt, and pepper. Bake until crispy.

Baked Sweet Potato Fries

Ingredients: Sweet potatoes, olive oil, paprika, salt, and pepper.

Instructions: Cut sweet potatoes into fries. Toss with olive oil, paprika, salt, and pepper. Bake until crispy.

Recipe 88

Frozen Grapes

Ingredients: Grapes.

Instructions: Freeze grapes for a refreshing snack.

Recipe 89

Pistachios

Ingredients: Pistachios.

Instructions: Enjoy pistachios as a healthy snack.

Recipe 90

Frozen Banana Bites

Ingredients: Banana slices, almond butter, dark chocolate.

Instructions: Spread almond butter on banana slices. Sandwich two slices together and dip in melted dark chocolate. Freeze until chocolate sets.

Cottage Cheese with Pineapple

Ingredients: Cottage cheese, diced pineapple.

Instructions: Mix cottage cheese with diced pineapple.

Rice Paper Veggie Rolls

Ingredients: Rice paper wrappers, mixed veggies (carrots, cucumbers, bell peppers, avocado), fresh basil leaves, low-sodium soy sauce.

Instructions: Soak rice paper wrappers in warm water until pliable. Fill with veggies and basil leaves. Roll tightly and serve with soy sauce for dipping.

Apple Slices with Cinnamon

Ingredients: Apple slices, ground cinnamon.

Instructions: Sprinkle apple slices with ground cinnamon.

Recipe 94

Greek Yogurt with Berries and Nuts

Ingredients: Greek yogurt, mixed berries, chopped almonds.

Instructions: Top Greek yogurt with berries and almonds.

Desserts

Recipe 95

Baked Apples with Cinnamon

Ingredients: Apples, ground cinnamon, honey.

Instructions: Core the apples and sprinkle with cinnamon. Drizzle with honey and bake until tender.

Recipe 96

Chia Seed Pudding

Ingredients: Chia seeds, almond milk, honey, mixed berries.

Instructions: Mix chia seeds, almond milk, and honey. Let it sit in the refrigerator until it thickens. Top with mixed berries before serving.

Recipe 97

Frozen Banana Ice Cream

Ingredients: Frozen bananas, almond milk, vanilla extract.

Instructions: Blend frozen bananas with almond milk and vanilla extract until creamy. Serve as ice cream.

Recipe 98

Coconut Date Balls

Ingredients: Dates, shredded coconut, almond flour, vanilla extract.

Instructions: Blend dates, coconut, almond flour, and vanilla extract in a food processor. Form into balls and refrigerate.

Recipe 99

Baked Peaches with Greek Yogurt

Ingredients: Peaches, honey, Greek yogurt, chopped walnuts.

Instructions: Cut peaches in half and remove pits. Drizzle with honey and bake until tender. Serve with Greek yogurt and walnuts.

Recipe 100

Frozen Yogurt Bark

Ingredients: Greek yogurt, honey, mixed berries, shredded coconut.

Instructions: Mix Greek yogurt and honey. Spread on a baking sheet and top with berries and coconut. Freeze until set. Break into pieces and serve.

Recipe 101

Berry Sorbet

Ingredients: Mixed berries, honey, lemon juice.

Instructions: Blend berries, honey, and lemon juice until smooth. Freeze until firm.

Recipe 102

Oatmeal Banana Cookies

Ingredients: Mashed bananas, rolled oats, chopped walnuts, honey, cinnamon.

Instructions: Mix mashed bananas, oats, walnuts, honey, and cinnamon. Drop spoonfuls onto a baking sheet and bake until firm.

Recipe 103

Greek Yogurt Cheesecake Bites

Ingredients: Greek yogurt, cream cheese, honey, vanilla extract.

Instructions: Mix Greek yogurt, cream cheese, honey, and vanilla extract. Spoon into mini muffin cups and freeze until set.

Recipe 104

Frozen Mango Popsicles

Ingredients: Mango chunks, orange juice, honey.

Instructions: Blend mango and orange juice until smooth. Sweeten with honey. Pour into popsicle molds and freeze until solid.

Recipe 105

Dark Chocolate Dipped Strawberries

Ingredients: Fresh strawberries, dark chocolate.

Instructions: Melt dark chocolate and dip strawberries into it. Allow chocolate to set.

Cherry Almond Energy Bites

Ingredients: Dates, dried cherries, almond butter, shredded coconut.

Instructions: Blend dates, cherries, and almond butter in a food processor. Form into balls and roll in shredded coconut.

Pumpkin Spice Chia Pudding

Ingredients: Chia seeds, pumpkin puree, almond milk, maple syrup, pumpkin pie spice.

Instructions: Mix chia seeds, pumpkin puree, almond milk, maple syrup, and pumpkin pie spice. Let it sit in the refrigerator until it thickens.

Coconut Mango Rice Pudding

Ingredients: Cooked brown rice, canned coconut milk, diced mango, honey, shredded coconut.

Instructions: Mix rice, coconut milk, mango, and honey. Top with shredded coconut.

Recipe 109

Watermelon and Mint Salad

Ingredients: Watermelon cubes, fresh mint leaves, lime juice, honey.

Instructions: Mix watermelon, mint, lime juice, and honey in a bowl.

Recipe 110

Mixed Berry Crumble

Ingredients: Mixed berries, almond flour, oats, honey, coconut oil.

Instructions: Mix berries with honey and place in a baking dish. In a separate bowl, mix almond flour, oats, and coconut oil until crumbly. Sprinkle over the berries and bake until golden.

Recipe 111

Peanut Butter Banana Bites

Ingredients: Banana slices, peanut butter, chopped peanuts.

Instructions: Spread peanut butter on banana slices. Roll in chopped peanuts.

Recipe 112

Mango Coconut Chia Pudding

Ingredients: Chia seeds, canned coconut milk, diced mango, honey.

Instructions: Mix chia seeds, coconut milk, mango, and honey. Let it sit in the refrigerator until it thickens.

Recipe 113

Blueberry Almond Bars

Ingredients: Almond flour, dried blueberries, honey, almond butter.

Instructions: Mix almond flour, blueberries, honey, and almond butter. Press into a baking dish and bake until firm.

Recipe 114

Avocado Chocolate Mousse

Ingredients: Avocado, cocoa powder, honey, almond milk.

Instructions: Blend avocado, cocoa powder, honey, and almond milk until smooth and creamy.

NOTES

BOOK 5

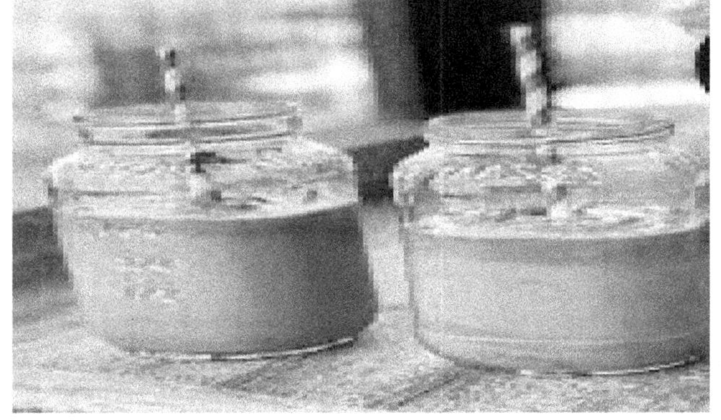

JUICE AND SMOOTHIES FOR RHEUMATOID ARTHRITIS, WITH PREPARATION INSTRUCTIONS

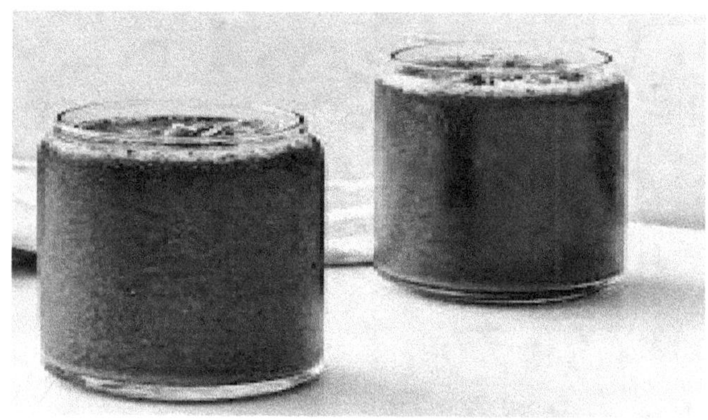

RHEUMATOID ARTHRITIS JUICE AND SMOOTHIES

Recipe 115

Carrot-Orange Juice

Ingredients: Carrots, oranges, ginger.

Instructions: Juice the carrots, oranges, and ginger together.

Recipe 116

Anti-Inflammatory Green Juice

Ingredients: Cucumber, celery, kale, parsley, lemon.

Instructions: Juice all the ingredients together.

Recipe 117

Beet-Apple Juice

Ingredients: Beets, apples, lemon.

Instructions: Juice the beets, apples, and lemon together.

Recipe 118

Pineapple-Turmeric Juice

Ingredients: Pineapple, turmeric root, lemon.

Instructions: Juice the pineapple, turmeric root, and lemon together.

Recipe 119

Ginger-Lemon Juice

Ingredients: Ginger, lemon, honey.

Instructions: Juice the ginger and lemon together. Sweeten with honey.

Recipe 120

Cucumber-Mint Juice

Ingredients: Cucumber, mint leaves, lime.

Instructions: Juice the cucumber and mint leaves together. Squeeze in lime juice.

Recipe 121

Watermelon-Cucumber Juice

Ingredients: Watermelon, cucumber, basil.

Instructions: Juice the watermelon and cucumber together. Garnish with fresh basil.

Strawberry-Beet Juice

Ingredients: Strawberries, beets, lime.

Instructions: Juice the strawberries and beets together. Squeeze in lime juice.

Spinach-Apple Juice

Ingredients: Spinach, apples, lemon.

Instructions: Juice the spinach, apples, and lemon together.

Blueberry-Pomegranate Juice

Ingredients: Blueberries, pomegranate seeds, lime.

Instructions: Juice the blueberries and pomegranate seeds together. Squeeze in lime juice.

Recipe 125

Orange-Ginger-Turmeric Juice

Ingredients: Oranges, ginger root, turmeric root.

Instructions: Juice the oranges, ginger root, and turmeric root together.

Recipe 126

Kale-Pineapple-Celery Juice

Ingredients: Kale, pineapple, celery, lemon.

Instructions: Juice the kale, pineapple, celery, and lemon together.

Recipe 127

Carrot-Apple-Ginger Juice

Ingredients: Carrots, apples, ginger root.

Instructions: Juice the carrots, apples, and ginger root together.

Recipe 128

Beet-Carrot-Orange Juice

Ingredients: Beets, carrots, oranges.

Instructions: Juice the beets, carrots, and oranges together.

Recipe 129

Lemon-Cucumber-Mint Juice

Ingredients: Lemon, cucumber, mint leaves.

Instructions: Juice the lemon, cucumber, and mint leaves together.

Recipe 130

Berry-Banana Smoothie

Ingredients: Mixed berries (strawberries, blueberries, raspberries), banana, Greek yogurt, almond milk.

Instructions: Blend all the ingredients until smooth.

Recipe 131

Green Power Smoothie

Ingredients: Spinach, kale, cucumber, green apple, lime, coconut water.

Instructions: Blend all the ingredients until smooth.

Recipe 132

Mango-Coconut Smoothie

Ingredients: Mango, canned coconut milk, Greek yogurt, honey.

Instructions: Blend all the ingredients until smooth.

Recipe 133

Pineapple-Ginger Smoothie

Ingredients: Pineapple, ginger root, Greek yogurt, almond milk.

Instructions: Blend all the ingredients until smooth.

Recipe 134

Peach-Turmeric Smoothie

Ingredients: Peaches, turmeric root, Greek yogurt, honey, almond milk.

Instructions: Blend all the ingredients until smooth.

Recipe 135

Blueberry-Spinach Smoothie

Ingredients: Blueberries, spinach, banana, Greek yogurt, almond milk.

Instructions: Blend all the ingredients until smooth.

Recipe 136

Strawberry-Kale Smoothie

Ingredients: Strawberries, kale, banana, Greek yogurt, coconut water.

Instructions: Blend all the ingredients until smooth.

Cherry-Almond Smoothie

Ingredients: Cherries, almond butter, Greek yogurt, honey, almond milk.

Instructions: Blend all the ingredients until smooth.

Mixed Berry-Avocado Smoothie

Ingredients: Mixed berries (strawberries, blueberries, raspberries), avocado, Greek yogurt, almond milk.

Instructions: Blend all the ingredients until smooth.

Orange-Carrot Smoothie

Ingredients: Oranges, carrots, banana, Greek yogurt, almond milk.

Instructions: Blend all the ingredients until smooth.

Recipe 140

Tropical Mango-Banana Smoothie

Ingredients: Mango, banana, coconut milk, Greek yogurt, honey.

Instructions: Blend all the ingredients until smooth.

Recipe 141

Spinach-Avocado Smoothie

Ingredients: Spinach, avocado, banana, Greek yogurt, coconut water.

Instructions: Blend all the ingredients until smooth.

Recipe 142

Raspberry-Almond Smoothie

Ingredients: Raspberries, almond butter, Greek yogurt, honey, almond milk.

Instructions: Blend all the ingredients until smooth.

Recipe 143

Kiwi-Pineapple Smoothie

Ingredients: Kiwi, pineapple, banana, Greek yogurt, coconut water.

Instructions: Blend all the ingredients until smooth.

Recipe 144

Pomegranate-Berry Smoothie

Ingredients: Pomegranate seeds, mixed berries (strawberries, blueberries, raspberries), Greek yogurt, almond milk.

Instructions: Blend all the ingredients until smooth.

Recipe 145

Beet-Berry Smoothie

Ingredients: Beets, mixed berries (strawberries, blueberries, raspberries), Greek yogurt, almond milk.

Instructions: Blend all the ingredients until smooth.

Recipe 146

Turmeric-Pineapple Smoothie

Ingredients: Pineapple, turmeric root, Greek yogurt, honey, coconut water.

Instructions: Blend all the ingredients until smooth.

Recipe 147

Mango-Banana-Avocado Smoothie

Ingredients: Mango, banana, avocado, Greek yogurt, almond milk.

Instructions: Blend all the ingredients until smooth.

Recipe 148

Peach-Raspberry Smoothie

Ingredients: Peaches, raspberries, Greek yogurt, honey, almond milk.

Instructions: Blend all the ingredients until smooth.

Recipe 149

Blueberry-Spinach-Avocado Smoothie

Ingredients: Blueberries, spinach, avocado, Greek yogurt, coconut water.

Instructions: Blend all the ingredients until smooth.

Recipe 150

Kale-Pineapple-Celery Juice

Ingredients: Kale, pineapple, celery, lemon.

Instructions: Juice the kale, pineapple, celery, and lemon together.

Please note: While recipes are made with anti-inflammatory ingredients, it is essential to consult with a healthcare professional or a registered dietitian before making significant changes to your diet, especially if you have specific dietary requirements or health conditions.

NOTES

CONCLUSION

Millions of people throughout the world suffer with rheumatoid arthritis, a chronic inflammatory disease that causes pain, stiffness, and swelling in the joints. Rheumatoid arthritis cannot be cured, but there are numerous strategies to treat and manage its symptoms, enhancing the quality of life for individuals who suffer from it.

Dietary changes are one of the most efficient strategies to manage rheumatoid arthritis. Adopting an anti-inflammatory diet, such as the DASH diet or the Mediterranean diet, can help to lessen joint discomfort and inflammation. These diets include a strong emphasis on complete, nutrient-dense foods, such as fresh produce, whole grains, lean meats, and healthy fats. Better rheumatoid arthritis management may also result from avoiding processed meals, sweet drinks, and foods high in sodium.

Rheumatoid arthritis sufferers can also benefit from including regular exercise in their daily regimen. Low-impact exercises that don't put too much strain on the joints, including swimming, yoga, and tai chi, can assist increase joint flexibility, muscular strength, and general physical function.

Additionally, effective rheumatoid arthritis management requires maintaining hydration, obtaining enough sleep, and controlling stress. These lifestyle habits can have a favorable effect on the symptoms and development of the illness and are important for general health.

Additionally, collaborating closely with medical specialists like rheumatologists, physical therapists, and nutritionists can offer individualized treatment and direction for people with rheumatoid arthritis. In order to address specific requirements and conditions, they can assist in customizing treatment regimens and suggest suitable solutions.

BONUS 1

MEAL PLAN

Day 1:

Breakfast: Berry Smoothie with Spinach and Flaxseed

Lunch: Quinoa Salad with Chickpeas, Avocado, and Lemon-Tahini Dressing

Dinner: Baked Salmon with Roasted Vegetables (bell peppers, broccoli, and carrots)

Dessert: Greek Yogurt with Honey and Almonds

Snack: Carrot Sticks with Hummus

Day 2:

Breakfast: Oatmeal with Chia Seeds, Blueberries, and Almond Milk

Lunch: Lentil Soup with Kale and Turmeric

Dinner: Grilled Chicken Breast with Quinoa Pilaf and Steamed Green Beans

Dessert: Baked Apple with Cinnamon and Walnuts

Snack: Celery Sticks with Almond Butter

Day 3:

Breakfast: Spinach and Mushroom Omelette with Whole Grain Toast

Lunch: Greek Salad with Grilled Shrimp

Dinner: Vegetable Stir-Fry with Tofu over Brown Rice

Dessert: Mango Sorbet

Snack: Mixed Nuts and Dried Fruits

Day 4:

Breakfast: Smoothie Bowl with Mixed Berries, Banana, and Almond Butter

Lunch: Chickpea Salad with Cucumber, Tomato, and Feta Cheese

Dinner: Baked Cod with Roasted Brussels Sprouts and Sweet Potatoes

Dessert: Dark Chocolate Covered Strawberries

Snack: Sliced Bell Peppers with Guacamole

Day 5:

Breakfast: Greek Yogurt Parfait with Granola and Mixed Berries

Lunch: Turkey and Avocado Wrap with Whole Grain Tortilla

Dinner: Vegetable Curry with Brown Rice

Dessert: Banana Nice Cream with Almond Butter Drizzle

Snack: Rice Cakes with Avocado Slices

Day 6:

Breakfast: Quinoa Porridge with Coconut Milk, Almonds, and Dried Cranberries

Lunch: Spinach Salad with Grilled Chicken, Strawberries, and Balsamic Vinaigrette

Dinner: Lentil and Vegetable Stew

Dessert: Chia Seed Pudding with Mango Puree

Snack: Edamame Beans

Day 7:

Breakfast: Whole Grain Pancakes with Fresh Fruit and Maple Syrup

Lunch: Tuna Salad with Mixed Greens and Lemon-Tahini Dressing

Dinner: Grilled Vegetable and Chicken Skewers with Quinoa

Dessert: Berry Compote with Greek Yogurt

Snack: Trail Mix with Nuts, Seeds, and Dried Fruit

Day 8:

Breakfast: Overnight Oats with Almond Milk, Berries, and Pumpkin Seeds

Lunch: Quinoa and Black Bean Salad with Corn, Tomato, and Lime-Cilantro Dressing

Dinner: Grilled Swordfish with Asparagus and Quinoa Pilaf

Dessert: Pineapple Coconut Chia Pudding

Snack: Apple Slices with Almond Butter

Day 9:

Breakfast: Green Smoothie with Kale, Pineapple, Banana, and Coconut Water

Lunch: Mediterranean Chickpea and Eggplant Stew

Dinner: Turkey Meatballs with Zucchini Noodles and Marinara Sauce

Dessert: Mixed Berry Crisp with Oat Topping

Snack: Greek Yogurt with Honey and Pistachios

Day 10:

Breakfast: Whole Grain Toast with Smashed Avocado and Poached Eggs

Lunch: Caprese Salad with Fresh Mozzarella, Tomato, and Basil

Dinner: Baked Halibut with Roasted Brussels Sprouts and Quinoa

Dessert: Mango Coconut Rice Pudding

Snack: Sliced Cucumber with Hummus

Day 11:

Breakfast: Buckwheat Pancakes with Maple Syrup and Sliced Banana

Lunch: Lentil and Kale Salad with Roasted Squash and Balsamic Vinaigrette

Dinner: Chicken Stir-Fry with Broccoli, Bell Peppers, and Brown Rice

Dessert: Blueberry Almond Crumble Bars

Snack: Cottage Cheese with Pineapple Chunks

Day 12:

Breakfast: Smoothie Bowl with Acai, Banana, Granola, and Coconut Flakes

Lunch: Quinoa and Roasted Vegetable Wrap with Tahini Sauce

Dinner: Grilled Salmon with Steamed Asparagus and Wild Rice

Dessert: Raspberry Lemon Sorbet

Snack: Rice Cakes with Cashew Butter

Day 13:

Breakfast: Chia Seed Breakfast Pudding with Almond Milk, Berries, and Almonds

Lunch: Greek Orzo Salad with Cherry Tomatoes, Cucumber, and Feta Cheese

Dinner: Vegetable and Chickpea Curry with Basmati Rice

Dessert: Chocolate Avocado Mousse

Snack: Mixed Berries with Greek Yogurt

Day 14:

Breakfast: Spinach and Feta Frittata with Whole Grain Toast

Lunch: Turkey and Quinoa Stuffed Bell Peppers

Dinner: Baked Cod with Lemon-Herb Quinoa and Roasted Cauliflower

Dessert: Coconut Mango Nice Cream

Snack: Almond Trail Mix

Day 15:

Breakfast: Berry Protein Smoothie with Spinach and Almond Milk

Lunch: Mediterranean Hummus Plate with Pita Bread, Olives, and Veggies

Dinner: Grilled Chicken Caesar Salad with Romaine Lettuce and Parmesan Cheese

Dessert: Peach and Raspberry Cobbler

Snack: Sliced Bell Peppers with Guacamole

Day 16:

Breakfast: Buckwheat Porridge with Mixed Berries and Almond Butter

Lunch: Quinoa Salad with Roasted Vegetables and Lemon-Tahini Dressing

Dinner: Baked Chicken Thighs with Sweet Potato Mash and Steamed Green Beans

Dessert: Greek Yogurt with Honey and Walnuts

Snack: Carrot Sticks with Hummus

Day 17:

Breakfast: Green Smoothie with Spinach, Pineapple, Banana, and Coconut Water

Lunch: Lentil Soup with Kale and Turmeric

Dinner: Grilled Salmon with Quinoa Pilaf and Roasted Brussels Sprouts

Dessert: Baked Apple with Cinnamon and Almonds

Snack: Celery Sticks with Almond Butter

Day 18:

Breakfast: Whole Grain Toast with Smashed Avocado, Tomato, and Poached Eggs

Lunch: Chickpea Salad with Cucumber, Tomato, Feta Cheese, and Lemon Vinaigrette

Dinner: Vegetable Stir-Fry with Tofu over Brown Rice

Dessert: Mango Sorbet

Snack: Mixed Nuts and Dried Fruits

Day 19:

Breakfast: Oatmeal with Chia Seeds, Blueberries, and Almond Milk

Lunch: Greek Salad with Grilled Shrimp

Dinner: Turkey Meatballs with Zucchini Noodles and Marinara Sauce

Dessert: Dark Chocolate Covered Strawberries

Snack: Sliced Bell Peppers with Hummus

Day 20:

Breakfast: Smoothie Bowl with Mixed Berries, Banana, Almond Butter, and Granola

Lunch: Caprese Salad with Fresh Mozzarella, Tomato, Basil, and Balsamic Glaze

Dinner: Baked Halibut with Roasted Asparagus and Quinoa

Dessert: Berry Compote with Greek Yogurt

Snack: Rice Cakes with Avocado Slices

Day 21:

Breakfast: Greek Yogurt Parfait with Granola and Mixed Berries

Lunch: Quinoa and Black Bean Salad with Corn, Tomato, and Lime-Cilantro Dressing

Dinner: Lentil and Vegetable Stew

Dessert: Banana Nice Cream with Almond Butter Drizzle

Snack: Edamame Beans

Day 22:

Breakfast: Spinach and Mushroom Omelette with Whole Grain Toast

Lunch: Mediterranean Hummus Plate with Pita Bread, Olives, and Veggies

Dinner: Grilled Chicken Breast with Roasted Sweet Potatoes and Steamed Broccoli

Dessert: Chia Seed Pudding with Mango Puree

Snack: Almond Trail Mix

Day 23:

Breakfast: Buckwheat Pancakes with Maple Syrup and Sliced Banana

Lunch: Turkey and Avocado Wrap with Whole Grain Tortilla

Dinner: Vegetable Curry with Brown Rice

Dessert: Coconut Mango Rice Pudding

Snack: Cottage Cheese with Pineapple Chunks

Day 24:

Breakfast: Overnight Oats with Almond Milk, Berries, and Chia Seeds

Lunch: Spinach Salad with Grilled Chicken, Strawberries, Almonds, and Balsamic Vinaigrette

Dinner: Grilled Vegetable and Chicken Skewers with Quinoa

Dessert: Raspberry Lemon Sorbet

Snack: Apple Slices with Almond Butter

Day 25:

Breakfast: Green Smoothie Bowl with Kale, Banana, Peanut Butter, and Granola

Lunch: Tuna Salad with Mixed Greens, Cherry Tomatoes, and Lemon-Tahini Dressing

Dinner: Baked Cod with Lemon-Herb Quinoa and Roasted Cauliflower

Dessert: Peach and Raspberry Cobbler

Snack: Greek Yogurt with Honey and Walnuts

Day 26:

Breakfast: Buckwheat Porridge with Mixed Berries, Almonds, and Maple Syrup

Lunch: Lentil and Kale Salad with Roasted Squash, Feta Cheese, and Balsamic Vinaigrette

Dinner: Chicken Stir-Fry with Broccoli, Bell Peppers, and Brown Rice

Dessert: Dark Chocolate Covered Strawberries

Snack: Carrot Sticks with Hummus

Day 27:

Breakfast: Whole Grain Toast with Smashed Avocado, Tomato, and Poached Eggs

Lunch: Greek Orzo Salad with Cucumber, Cherry Tomatoes, Feta Cheese, and Lemon Vinaigrette

Dinner: Vegetable and Chickpea Curry with Basmati Rice

Dessert: Blueberry Almond Crumble Bars

Snack: Celery Sticks with Almond Butter

Day 28:

Breakfast: Smoothie Bowl with Acai, Banana, Mixed Berries, Granola, and Coconut Flakes

Lunch: Quinoa and Roasted Vegetable Wrap with Hummus

Dinner: Baked Chicken Thighs with Sweet Potato Mash and Steamed Green Beans

Dessert: Coconut Mango Nice Cream

Snack: Mixed Nuts and Dried Fruits

BONUS 2

SHOPPING GUIDE TAILORED FOR RHEUMATOID ARTHRITIS

Produce:

Leafy greens (spinach, kale, Swiss chard)

Berries (blueberries, strawberries, raspberries)

Cruciferous vegetables (broccoli, cauliflower, Brussels sprouts)

Colorful vegetables (bell peppers, carrots, sweet potatoes)

Citrus fruits (oranges, lemons, limes)

Avocados

Tomatoes

Garlic

Onions

Whole Grains:

Quinoa

Brown rice

Oats

Whole wheat bread and pasta

Barley

Buckwheat

Millet

Proteins:

Fatty fish (salmon, mackerel, sardines)

Lean poultry (chicken, turkey)

Tofu

Beans and legumes (lentils, chickpeas, black beans)

Nuts and seeds (almonds, walnuts, chia seeds, flaxseeds)

Dairy and Alternatives:

Greek yogurt

Cottage cheese

Almond milk

Soy milk

Coconut milk

Healthy Fats:

Extra virgin olive oil

Avocado oil

Coconut oil

Nuts (almonds, walnuts, pistachios)

Seeds (chia seeds, flaxseeds, pumpkin seeds)

Herbs and Spices:

Turmeric

Ginger

Cinnamon

Rosemary

Basil

Oregano

Thyme

Condiments:

Balsamic vinegar

Apple cider vinegar

Mustard (preferably Dijon)

Tahini

Hummus

Others:

Green tea

Dark chocolate (70% cocoa or higher)

Honey

Herbal teas (such as chamomile or peppermint)

Whole grain snacks (rice cakes, popcorn)

Tips for Shopping

Choose fresh, whole foods over processed ones whenever possible.

Opt for organic produce to minimize exposure to pesticides.

Read labels carefully and avoid foods with additives, preservatives, and artificial ingredients.

Incorporate a variety of colors into your diet to ensure a wide range of nutrients.

Buy frozen fruits and vegetables as they are often just as nutritious as fresh and can be more convenient.

Experiment with different herbs and spices to add flavor to your meals without relying on excessive salt or sugar.

By following this shopping guide and incorporating these foods into your diet regularly, you can help support your overall health and manage the symptoms of Rheumatoid Arthritis.

Can you imagine the freedom of enjoying a delicious meal without worrying about the consequences? This cookbook unlocks that freedom, empowering you to:

Reduce inflammation and manage RA flare-ups
Boost your energy levels and feel empowered
Take back control of your health and well-being

Don't miss out! RA doesn't have to steal another flavorful bite. This cookbook is your solution to delicious, anti-inflammatory relief.

Order your copy right away and reclaim your kitchen, your health, and your joy for food!